THE BODY'S ROLE IN
ADDICTIONS

THE BODY'S ROLE IN
ADDICTIONS

Jean Armour

BALBOA.
PRESS

A DIVISION OF HAY HOUSE

Balboa Press books may be ordered through booksellers or by contacting:

Balboa Press
A Division of Hay House
1663 Liberty Drive
Bloomington, IN 47403
www.balboapress.com
1-(877) 407-4847

Because of the dynamic nature of the Internet, any web addresses or
links contained in this book may have changed since publication and
may no longer be valid. The views expressed in this work are solely those
of the author and do not necessarily reflect the views of the publisher,
and the publisher hereby disclaims any responsibility for them.

The author of this book does not dispense medical advice or prescribe the use
of any technique as a form of treatment for physical, emotional, or medical
problems without the advice of a physician, either directly or indirectly. The
intent of the author is only to offer information of a general nature to help
you in your quest for emotional and spiritual well-being. In the event you use
any of the information in this book for yourself, which is your constitutional
right, the author and the publisher assume no responsibility for your actions.

Certain stock imagery © Thinkstock.
Any people depicted in stock imagery provided by Thinkstock are
models, and such images are being used for illustrative purposes only.

ISBN: 978-1-4525-4757-2 (e)
ISBN: 978-1-4525-4758-9 (sc)

Library of Congress Control Number: 2012902753

Printed in the United States of America

Balboa Press rev. date: 3/16/2012

CONTENTS

INTRODUCTION

Writing a book was not something I intended as one of my life goals. Writing seems tedious, putting on paper what easily flows from one's mouth is laborious, time consuming and, in some ways, artificial. Standing in front of a group of people who have designated themselves as learners is wonderful. The connection between people is really the learning vehicle and the exchange of knowledge, life experience and wisdom is what binds us together as fellow travelers throughout our lives.

But, I have written a book. Those responsible for this change in life goals have been the combined efforts of wonderful friends, eager students who requested that I put on paper what I taught in class, and the loving support of dear family members. For their belief in me, and what I had to offer, I am deeply touched and grateful.

The biggest stumbling block about getting started in such a venture was the concern that there was nothing new to write. The dedicated researchers, professional writers, and self-help authors have contributed volumes from which any avid learner can choose for a rainy day activity with an apple and the ambiance of a glowing fireplace, or a serious perusal in the local library or study hall. What do I have to add to the mix?

My students have said their reason for asking for a book was my apparent ability to study the great works of researchers and 'bring it all together' in an understandable format for lay persons and counselors who either are not interested in pouring through the literature, have difficulty with the jargon, or simply are too busy to gather all that knowledge from the various sources available.

For some unknown reason, gathering the knowledge has been fun for me, and a life quest. I am clearly stating that I am not a researcher, but I am a clinician in the Human Service fields with combined experience as a nurse, licensed therapist, trainer, adjunct professor, executive manager, and consultant. Years of experience alone do not necessarily mean that wisdom has accrued or that skill has been developed.

However, that can be the outcome of one's life experiences, and my hope is that in the following pages I will be able to meet the expectation for something of value to appear.

These pages are not designed as a college text or medical primer. It is scaled down in technical information, but hopefully correct in the concepts which are intended to be helpful for the reader. Analogies are used which can help the reader add this new information to something that is already part of their life experience. Hopefully, this approach will create a learning style that makes sense, is easy to understand, and remember. It is also not intended to deal with the impact of individual substances and their particular effect in the body. Rather, understanding how the body is structured and functions allows for a broader understanding of the reason for the symptoms that are noticed when substances have been used.

I have been a teacher. I am the product of teachers and mentors from whom I have learned. Some of them are not aware of the impact they have had on my life, and to each of them I owe a debt of gratitude for their role in forming not only who I am today, but also what I have to share with you, the reader. The list is lengthy and begins many years ago when I was not thinking of teaching at all. I was involved in all the activities of family life and aware that I needed to begin my search for meaning on the inside of me. That learning laid the foundation for exploring my world on the outside, and finding a place where I had a niche and something to share that would make a difference. This book represents that learning and is given as a gift in the hopes that as you read you will further your awareness of the gifts you have to share with your fellow travelers. Blessings to each one.

CHAPTER 1

The Body

If the measure of effectiveness in any Human Services related field is the outcome in client care, the substance abuse treatment field has been sadly ineffective for many of those seeking our help. Clearly there are those who have made significant strides in overcoming the impact that the use of addicting chemicals has had in their lives. I applaud them for their persistence and great personal achievement. There are others who have gone to the same treatment programs, attended the same Twelve Step meetings, read the same books, talked with the same counselors and have not been able, up to this point, to achieve the same success.

Blaming is an unproductive way of skirting the issue of how we can develop skill in effectively relating to those asking for assistance in achieving sobriety. Perhaps one of the contributing factors in our lack of success has been our lack of understanding about the body, how substances affect the body, and what can be done to cooperate with the body's wisdom for healing. What we have gleaned from the combined efforts of researchers, counselors, medical personnel and writers is that the body is truly a marvelous 'piece of work'.

From the initial combining of the ovum and sperm, which sets in place an internal clock that will orchestrate the timing of developmental tasks and lays the architectural blueprint for the unfolding of the body and all its related functions, to the maintaining of life and making the necessary repairs as we experience the bumps of illnesses, toxins, accidents, and poor nutrition, our body has the internal wisdom to be successful. Our job is to discover the body's wisdom, follow its lead in the healing process, and provide the support it requires for success.

The body is designed in a simple, yet complex way. It begins with building blocks and then creates the structure that houses our sense of self, very much like a child with blocks who designs towers, houses, and forts. The building block of the body is the *cell*. For our purposes we will think of the cell as a circle with a membrane attached to its outer edge. There are little doors, called receptors, which allow the exchange of certain nutrients into the cell and carries away waste products no longer needed. Part of the role of the membrane is to provide protection for the cell in the form of monitoring what is allowed in, and to keep in place nutrients the cell must have to function. Cell membranes are made from the fat that we eat (more about that later), and their health influences the health of the cell and its ability to perform its specialized duties.

The architectural design, or blueprint for the body, is encoded in the DNA and housed in each cell. When cells that perform the same function in the body join together, they create an *organ*. Some examples of organs include the heart, lungs, liver, spleen, gall bladder and large intestine. When organs join together to perform specific functions a *system* is created.

The gastrointestinal system is a combination of many organs working together to perform the task of handling food. The steps of eating food, breaking it down into small particles, processing it into a form that the body can use, passing it along a conveyor belt so the nutrients can be absorbed into the nearby capillaries, reabsorbing water back into the blood stream from the leftovers that were not used, and then holding the remains until it is convenient to dump them can be seen as the combined efforts of the organs in this system of the body. There are other systems. The genitourinary system processes liquid wastes from the body, the respiratory system handles breathing, and the circulatory system has the responsibility to transport both nutrients and waste products throughout the body.

There are seven systems in all and when they join together the body is created. At each level the membranes are hard at work. There are membranes covering the organs, the systems, and the body. The membrane for the body is the skin, which has the same protective function as the membrane around the smallest cell, to keep the contents of the body (cell) intact, to allow certain things to pass across the skin, and to keep out things that would be harmful.

Each cell knows what it needs to complete its task in the body and will be selective as it notices various raw materials passing by in the capillaries. It is not unlike going to a cafeteria with our tray and picking what we are interested in eating for that meal. The cell will select the raw materials it needs and allow others to pass along to a neighboring cell that will select different materials for its needs. The wisdom of the cell in knowing what it needs is baffling. As it is watching the parade of nutrients, waiting for what it needs, it may be alarmed to discover there is nothing on the line it needs today. There may need to be a reconsideration of what it is looking for and Plan B may be instituted, adapting to what is available, not what is preferred. Of course, that also means that the health and function of the cell has also shifted to Plan B status (or maybe F or J).

We'll talk more about the role of nutrition starting in Chapter 8, but at the moment it is enough to say that Nature's way of providing the cells, organs, systems and body with the raw materials it needs is through the foods we eat on a daily basis. Just like our car would not run very well on paint thinner or kerosene, our bodies begin to sputter when the raw materials we need are not provided.

More sputtering happens when toxins are taken into the body. Those might come in the form of environmental chemicals such as lead, mercury, aluminum, and bug spray. Or, they might come in the form of addicting chemicals such as alcohol, tobacco, methamphetamine, or heroin. The body isn't set up to select any of these chemicals in the cafeteria line as preferred materials, and in fact, if the selection is made, some disastrous results can follow. Some of these chemicals fool the cell into selecting them because they look like the real thing, or are at least close enough to cause confusion, so they get selected any way. Once they enter the cell, alarms can go off, sending messages out to all the cell members that a change in plans is required to adjust to this situation. We'll talk more about these changes and the chaos created in the body as we move through our time together.

At the same time that the body cells and tissues are being affected by whatever we have taken in, it is figuring out a way to deal with the situation. There are four basic steps in handling substances that the body is exposed to. The first step is *absorption*. It simply means the method of getting something from the outside into the body. There are many ways to accomplish this, including over the skin, through the mouth and intestinal tract, across any membrane, into the lungs, and with the use of needles.

The slowest route is by passing over the skin barrier. This is slow because the substance has to cross several layers of skin tissue, enter the small capillaries, be taken up into the small veins called venules, then into the larger veins, through the liver, off to the heart, to the lungs, back to the heart, then to the brain. Whew! That is quite a trip which involves many depots along the way and the loss of some of its potency as well. For example, a person might be caught with LSD microdots in their hand and if they close their hand they will absorb the drug through the skin in the order described and will experience a drug effect. There will not be an immediate drug 'rush' experience however.

Chemicals taken orally through the mouth will meet with the hydrochloric acid and the digestive enzymes in the gastrointestinal system which are necessary for processing food. The chemical will be broken down, passed into the blood vessels, off to the liver and then the same order of heart, lungs, heart, and the final destination of the brain response to the chemical. The speed of a drug effect from a substance taken orally depends on several things, one of which is whether or not there is food in the stomach. In general there is at least a twenty to thirty minute delay before there is a noticeable drug effect.

All openings to the outside of the body are lined with a membrane which secretes a fluid known as mucous. The role of the fluid is to keep the tissue moist so it can perform its functions. When it dries out, the result is similar to the unpleasant feeling you experience when your nose feels too dry, but more importantly, the function of the membrane is interfered with. There are small blood vessels called capillaries which draw chemicals touching the membranes into the larger blood vessels and then they join the usual trip to the brain. These membranes allow substances such as cocaine or heroin to be snorted into the nasal passages, suppositories can be inserted into the vagina if a woman has a yeast infection or inserted into the rectum if constipated (people also have stuffed marijuana leaves into that cavity). Chemicals have also been put into the space between the lower eyelid and the eye known as the conjunctiva. Sometimes LSD has been used in this manner.

Needles can also be used to introduce substances into the body. The simplest way is inserting the needle right under the surface of the skin, often called 'skin popping'. There is no worry about getting into a vein, you just insert the needle and push the plunger to release the liquid. Many people begin their use of heroin in this manner, especially if they have old childhood feelings from the doctors' office of queasiness when they see a needle coming toward them. Another method of needle use is called intramuscular, or IM. It is directed at more of a vertical angle and injects the liquid into a muscle from which it will be absorbed into the surrounding blood vessels. The more common method of needle use for substance abusers is injecting directly into the veins, often called 'slamming' or 'mainlining'.

Inhalation is the fastest way to experience a drug effect because the substance is already in the lungs. It only needs to travel back to the heart and then to the brain. That trip takes about seven (7) seconds. This is one of the reasons that it is difficult to stop smoking. The drug reward is immediate and intense, since it does not need to go through the liver first, picking up enzymes which begin the breakdown process and reducing the intensity of the drug effect.

People who use addicting chemicals will often 'graduate' to using the IV method because the entire syringe full of substance is delivered to the brain at one time making the experience more intense than taking several puffs of a cigarette, a crack pipe or marijuana joint over a period of several minutes.

An assessment of chemical use includes questions about how the substance is taken into the body, since the answer provides information about the severity of the use problem as well as potential risk factors that might be present due to sharing their 'works' (syringes and needles) with other users who may have blood borne diseases such as HIV or various forms of hepatitis.

The second step in the process of handling a chemical is called *distribution*. It literally means how the substance circulates throughout the body rather than staying at the site of ingestion. The primary way in which this happens is through the arteries, veins and capillary system. It's rather like a road trip where the chemical goes zooming around, stopping at various organs and affecting its function in some way. Another system which can be involved in the distribution of a chemical is known as the lymph system. Its primary role has to do with fighting infection and catching germs in the specialized traps known as nodes so they do not exit on the other side and continue to spread throughout the body. They are located in places like the armpits, the groin, and the sides of the neck, and are usually swollen when we have an infection. They can often be felt if you run your fingers over those areas when you are sick.

The tonsils are also lymph nodes, or germ traps, and medical practice many years ago included removing tonsils from children at about five years of age to prevent tonsillitis problems later. Now we know that is not the best idea. Nature put them there for a reason, so the old trip to the operating room, having an unpleasant experience with ether and a very sore throat after the experience, is not the preferred approach. Even with the promise of ice cream after surgery, many people remember that as an unpleasant childhood experience.

After taking a substance in and letting it roam around in the body through the circulatory and lymph systems, the next step is changing it in some way. It clearly can't stay in the form in which it was taken in. It needs to be used or gotten rid of. In the use of addictive chemicals, medications, and all sorts of toxins, the body figures out a way to change the substance so it can be removed from the body. The technical term for this process is *metabolism*. Metabolism really has two processes: one builds up (anabolism) and the other breaks substances down (catabolism). Here we are interested in the breakdown process, but for clarity we will simply call it metabolism. There is a special organ in the body which has the primary responsibility to take something potentially harmful and convert it into a harmless substance so it can be eliminated from the body. That miracle worker is the liver.

The liver is located under the right side of the rib cage, is burgundy in color, about eight inches across, six inches deep and three quarters of an inch thick. It looks pretty much like the liver you see at the grocery store, for those of you who like liver and onions. Believe it or not, there are people who grew up on that food dish and relish it. There are others for whom the very mention of liver causes a nauseous response. The liver has several jobs to do, one of which is to change a potentially harmful substance that somehow got into the body so it loses its ability to be destructive.

We can use alcohol as an easy example since the metabolism process is pretty simple. For anyone, whether they have a problem with the use of alcohol or not, when alcohol enters the body, the liver is alerted that there is something there that is potentially harmful and needs to be changed so it can be eliminated. The liver responds by producing an enzyme called *alcohol dehydrogenase* to begin the process. The enzyme interacts with the alcohol and converts it to the first stage of breakdown which is called *acetaldehyde.* We call this a metabolite, from the process of metabolism, which basically means that the body made it from the parent product, alcohol. It is the acetaldehyde which causes people to feel nauseated, their pulse to race, and their face to be flushed. The liver then produces another enzyme, this time called *acetaldehyde dehydrogenase*, which changes the acetaldehyde by breaking it down to acetic acid (vinegar), then on to carbon dioxide, which we breathe out, and water, which is eliminated primarily through the kidneys. At this point the process is complete and the chemical no longer has the potential for harming the body.

In review:

> Alcohol
> Alcohol dehydrogenase (an enzyme)
> Acetaldehyde (a metabolite)
> Acetaldehyde dehydrogenase (an enzyme)
> Acetic acid (vinegar)
> Carbon dioxide & water

All drugs are broken down in this way whether prescribed as a pharmaceutical product or a 'street' drug. Different enzymes are produced and differing metabolites are created, but the process is similar for each drug. Alcohol is a very simple process, whereas other drugs may have a more complex breakdown process and require a longer time to achieve completion of the process. When urine specimens are 'positive' if monitoring for substance use, it is the metabolite that is picked up in the urine since usually there has been a time lag between use and obtaining the specimen.

After the metabolism process is complete the body needs to get rid of the end products, which is called *elimination*. For most substances that are abused, elimination is done primarily through the kidneys, with two exceptions: Methadone is eliminated primarily through sweat, and LSD is eliminated primarily through the feces. Small amounts of the end products are also eliminated through the sweat, breath, skin and hair (which is why breathalyzers and other forms of testing work).

So... when a potentially toxic substance is taken into the body, a process is set in motion to render the substance harmless and get rid of it as quickly as possible. It's a miraculous way of dealing with emergencies and maintaining the body's state of equilibrium, or being 'normal'.

CHAPTER 2

Half-Life and the Continuum

The speed with which the body can deal with these emergencies is partly based on something we call 'half-life'. We're used to thinking of half-life being connected to metals such as uranium or plutonium, however all substances of abuse have a half-life as well. An easy definition is 'the amount of time it takes for half of the molecules to be removed from the blood stream' (not the body). It is the job of the liver to oversee this process and produce the necessary enzymes.

Some substances love fat and can attach to fat cells resulting in no effect of the drug on the body (no continuing high), and no breakdown or metabolism either. Marijuana is a good example of this. In these cases, anything that causes the breakdown of fat can release some of the un-metabolized drug back into the blood stream, causing either a mild drug effect or showing up in a drug test as being 'hot', 'dirty' or 'positive'. Some examples of fat breakdown might include being sick, beginning an exercise program, sitting in a sauna, or going on a diet.

Here's how half-life works. We'll use methadone as the example, however all drugs follow a similar pattern. What is different for each drug is the speed with which this process happens. If we begin with sixteen (16) molecules of methadone, in twenty four hours (which is the half-life for methadone) half of the molecules are broken down, leaving eight (8). In another twenty four hours half of the remaining molecules are broken down, leaving four (4), within the next twenty four hours we are down to two (2), and then one (1) in another twenty four hour period. The general guideline is that it takes five (5) half-lives to eliminate a substance from the blood stream at least to the point where it is difficult to detect in a lab specimen. There are exceptions such as how healthy the liver is, how much substance a person took into their body during a short period of time, or if there was an extended period of excessive use.

In general, half-life times can be designated as short, medium or long. Even though information is available about more specific half-lives, memorizing that data is probably not that important. What is useful is having an idea about which of the three categories the drug falls within, so a prediction can be made about when a drug test must be done if the substance is to be detected.

Another useful guideline is that the half-life can also predict how often the person may want to re-dose since the drug effect will be waning. This is not always reliable as a measuring stick, however, since the effect of the drug may not line up accurately with the half-life. An example is cocaine. The half-life for cocaine is about two to four (2-4) hours; however the drug effect is only eight to twenty minutes for someone who smokes crack or mainlines. The person using cocaine will feel great for about a twenty minute period and then begin a rapid decline in mood and will want to re-dose. It doesn't take long for several doses to pile up before the first dose has even begun the breakdown process.

Pharmaceutical drugs also have a half-life about which you can get information by asking the pharmacist in any of the many locations which dispense pharmaceutical medications. An interesting piece of information which may help you to be more conscientious about taking prescribed medicines is that how often you are asked to take a new dose, (every 4, 6, 8 hours, etc.), is based on half-life. A new dose is needed that often to keep the blood level up at the desired level. If we forget to take the medicine bottle to work with us and the blood level drops too low before we get back home and take the next dose, the effectiveness of the medicine will be diminished.

How often an addicting substance is taken into the body has effects much beyond blood level effects for a prescribed medication. In the chemical dependency field, we know that repeated doses can result in internal adjustments which can have long term effects and create a dependency on the substance. In fact, from a clinician's point of view, an accurate assessment of the extent of the usage is needed to provide guidance about how to proceed with a treatment regime.

In far too many clinics, the same treatment programming is applied to all clients without consideration for their particular reason for beginning the use, or the degree to which internal adjustments have reset what is considered 'normal'. More about that later.

Not everyone who uses a mind altering substance develops a problem with its use. There is a continuum which defines whether or not there are concerns that may have developed. The first stage of the continuum is *use*. Many, in fact most, people who use alcohol fit into this category. They may drink on a regular basis, a glass of wine for dinner every evening, or at a special occasion or event. The criteria used to determine if people fit into this category is that there are NO harmful consequences. No *Driving Under the Influence* (DUI), accident, Domestic Violence citation or physical problems. The guideline for the use of alcohol with no body tissue damage is generally accepted to be for adult males two drinks per day and for adult females one to one and a half drinks per day. A 'drink' is considered to be a can of beer, 4 ounces of wine, or a shot of whiskey.

The second level of the continuum is *misuse*. In this situation there is a legitimate reason to use a substance, but if it is used inappropriately, there are consequences. A common example is the misuse of antibiotics. If you have strep throat and the doctor prescribes an antibiotic, you most often will have a ten day supply. The reason for the ten day supply is that the streptococcus is a persistent little critter and after weakening it, the antibiotic still needs to be taken until it finally gives up and dies. There are more potent antibiotics with only a few doses needed but in many (if not most) cases, it is due to earlier misuse which requires a more potent version to address the current infection.

It might go something like this: a person takes the antibiotic as prescribed until one day they forget their bottle of pills at home and miss a dose or two. So when they return home and begin taking them again, the blood level will have dropped and some of the intended effect now is lost and has to be regained. In that case, even when the bottle is empty, the offending microorganisms might not be completely destroyed.

Another scenario might be that the person faithfully takes the pills as prescribed until day seven when their throat no longer hurts, energy is restored and they consider themselves cured, so they stop taking their antibiotic. Then in a couple of weeks they may talk with their neighbor who complains that her throat was scratchy today and she just wanted to come home in the worst way. The person with the current prescription may say something like, 'just a minute', and run home and get their three day supply of antibiotics for the neighbor.

Now there are two people who have not destroyed the microorganisms, however, both of them have developed antibodies which work against antibiotics so that the next time they need an antibiotic they will not be as effective. This explains the need for the potent versions. There are many people who have created this problem for themselves due to the misuse of a legitimate drug. Prescription medications such as Valium, Percoset or sleeping pills could also be used inappropriately, resulting in some negative consequences.

The third continuum level is *abuse*. In this situation *there are <u>always</u> negative consequences.* They might include such things as legal problems, a *Driving Under the Influence* (DUI) arrest, a Domestic Violence citation, accidents, or physical problems such as ulcers, emphysema, cancer, or cirrhosis. Up to this point in the continuum what is NORMAL is <u>NO</u> substance in the body. A person might be sick while using, such as having a reddened face or a racing pulse rate with alcohol use, but the symptoms go away when they stop using the substance. Let's use alcohol as an example here.

When a person has a drink of alcohol, whether they have a problem with alcohol or not, the liver notices something in the body that is potentially harmful and immediately begins to put in place a plan of action to have the body go back to 'normal' - no alcohol in the body. The liver releases an enzyme which has the job of beginning the breakdown process. If drinking seems to be a steady occurrence the liver says to itself that it better have some enzyme standing by because at any moment some alcohol is likely to come along. Now, the person has to drink more to get the desired effect because the enzymes begin their work more quickly.

If this practice continues and the person is drinking more to offset the enzyme effect, the liver has another conversation with itself saying that it had earlier clearly underestimated the need and makes even more enzymes standing by to handle the soon expected alcohol. This chess match continues with the liver trying to protect the person, and the person needing to drink more to get the desired effect until finally the liver says 'I was wrong all along - what is normal is having alcohol (or heroin, cocaine, methamphetamine) in my body', and resets what normal is. Technically this process is called *enzyme induction*. It simply means that the liver is 'induced' to make additional enzymes in an attempt to deal with a situation that needs some resolution. Another term that is used is Tolerance, meaning the person can now tolerate larger and larger amounts of the substance.

Since the liver is the main player in this scenario, there are situations that may affect its ability to be efficient. It may be weakened in some way, through a form of hepatitis, cirrhosis, or other physical condition, or it may be preoccupied with dealing with other issues at the moment and not able to attend fully to the latest situation. The overall health of the liver, as well as the age of the person, both play a role. In general, the younger we are, the less accumulative stress has accrued and the easier it is for the liver to provide the protection needed in a new situation.

When the liver comes to the conclusion that it is normal to have the substance in the body, normal is reset and body tissue is changed to adapt to the presence of the substance. Now the body will complain when there isn't enough substance currently present in the body. We call this *withdrawal*. Withdrawal cannot happen until the body has reset normal; thus it is always an indicator that the person has now moved to another level on the continuum, *dependence*.

In assessing where a person might be on the continuum particular attention needs to be paid to determining if this line has been crossed. Let's use alcohol again as the example. If you go to a major concert, particularly outdoors, you will notice that the sheriff's officers are standing at the exit watching to see if people enjoyed the concert a little too much. If they suspect that has happened, they invite the person to get into their vehicle and take them to a detoxification facility. The staff will need to assess for abuse or dependence, since that will help determine the level of care needed and the potential for life threatening problems to occur.

If the person is an abuser of alcohol, when the staff asks them to blow into the breathalyzer the reading will be elevated, and the pulse and blood pressure readings will be elevated as well. This is because the body is not feeling normal. As the alcohol leaves their body, both sets of readings will go down and return to their normal settings and the person will be safe to leave the facility. They will not be sick after leaving.

Exactly the opposite is true if a person is dependent. For this person the breathalyzer readings will be elevated, sometimes very high, but the pulse and blood pressure may not be very elevated because this state of intoxication is now the norm. For this person, as the blood alcohol level goes down, the body begins to complain and the vital signs (the pulse, blood pressure, respirations, and temperature) may begin to elevate dramatically. This person can be at risk for life threatening problems such as grand mal seizures, cardiac arrest, or respiratory arrest.

A dependent person is not safe to leave the facility as soon as they blow a 0.000 BAL (Blood Alcohol Level). If they leave at this time there are two options, to be sick by themselves in the community, or to drink again so their body will feel that normal has been restored. Many people leave too soon and some are readmitted that same day or in the near future because they leave and resume their drinking to avoid the withdrawal process.

A later stage of dependency is referred to as *addiction* in which case the craving is intensified following the withdrawal. Tobacco is a good example here. If a person is dependent on tobacco and goes through the withdrawal experience successfully, there may not be a lot of misery later when they smell someone else smoking, desperately wishing they could smoke again themselves. In fact, they may take the situation lightly and assume that they could begin again and still quit easily, perhaps thinking that they 'have a better constitution than other people'. What they will discover, however, if they do that a time or two, is that they will increase their discomfort in the withdrawal process and there can be considerable discomfort long after their last cigarette, called craving. There are people who haven't had a cigarette in many years, and for some of them, hardly a day goes by that they don't wish they could have one.

Labeling a person as an abuser or dependent and using that as a pressure point to achieve guilt or shame is not helpful in their decision making about whether they need or want to do something about their use of a substance. Labeling is most helpful for the clinician to guide the treatment decisions and to be prepared to handle withdrawal difficulties as they occur. When the person using a substance labels themselves, it often is an indicator of their awareness of the role that the substance plays in their life and may serve as a motivator to make the changes that will be difficult to achieve.

CHAPTER 3

Neurons

All these cells, organs and systems need a way of discussing matters with each other if they are to have a happy and well functioning community. This is directed by two primary systems in the body. The first is the circulatory system which is a complex highway department where substances like chemicals, foodstuff, and hormones travel to all points in the body and deliver their goods to the surrounding tissue. The circulatory system is composed of arteries, veins, and capillaries with the heart directing the flow of traffic.

Another important part of this communication system is called the nervous system. Even though the basic building block of the body is a cell, many of which are roundish in shape, there is a special name and shape for nerve cells which are called neurons. The neuron has several long projections rather like wavy arms that are connected to the middle part of the cell. These projections are called *Dendrites* and have many little openings called receptors which receive message chemicals into the neuron. The chemicals stimulate an electrical response which then travels into the interior of the cell called the *Cell Body*.

The Cell Body has a couple of jobs to do. One of its tasks is to house the DNA or blueprint of the genetic structure of the body and hold the architectural design for making a replacement for itself, called a daughter cell. Another task, the one we are focusing on, is providing for the eventuality that a message would need to be sent on to another cell. Its way of handling this is to produce a variety of chemicals which will serve to conduct the messages from one neuron to another. In all, there are approximately one hundred such chemicals that the neurons are capable of producing and distributing, however as we learn more about the body we will surely discover there are more. These chemicals have the common umbrella name of neurotransmitter and each of the chemicals have been christened with a name of their own, such as dopamine and serotonin.

These chemicals are produced, then travel down one long arm like projection called the *Axon* to its end points called *Nodes*. Inside the nodes there are many storage packets called *Vesicles* which are like little pantries and hold the neurotransmitters until they are needed. At that time, they are dumped out of the neuron into the surrounding space which is called the *Synapse*. It would be nice and less confusing if there were only one name for this space, but it has also been called the Synaptic Cleft, and the Synaptic Gap.

The signal to dump the neurotransmitters is an electrical charge which is created in the neuron by minerals such as sodium and potassium moving back and forth over the wall of the axon. The axon is covered by a fatty membrane called the *Myelin Sheath*. The health of the cell and the ability to create an electrical charge is largely dependent on the condition of the myelin and the types of fat we ingest into our bodies. We'll discuss this in more detail later.

As the electrical charge travels down the axon to the storage sites, or vesicles, the vesicles are stimulated by the electrical charge and move to the edge of the axon where they meld with the membrane, creating an opening so the neurotransmitters can be released into the synapse.

In the synaptic space there are no railroad tracks or roads to direct the traffic. In fact, the neurotransmitters are free to swim around. Some will go directly across the gap to another neuron and be invited into the receptor. Other neurotransmitters may be like adolescents and want to go exploring, so they swim off in various directions. According to Candice Pert, PhD, the receptors and the neurotransmitter both do a little dance which includes a humming sound, and the vibration can be called e-motion. Think about email being electronic mail and in a similar way, e-motion is electrical motion. The result is a feeling which we identify and can express. As the neurotransmitter and receptor vibrate they attract each other. The neurotransmitter can then be drawn into the receptor and the receiving neuron is activated. (Figure 1)

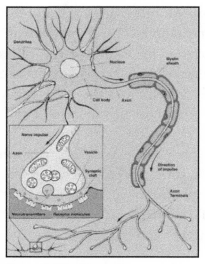

Figure 1. The Neuron
Photo courtesy of the NIDA Web site.

Each neurotransmitter and molecule has a corresponding shape and they are drawn to each other. That also means that molecules that aren't a match are not taken in. Pharmaceutical molecules which are created to mimic a natural substance, or drugs which are used for a mind altering effect, are also similar to the molecule the body designed. In fact, they are often a better fit into the receptor so might be selected in preference to the neurotransmitter if both are in the synapse at the same time. One problem created by this is that the stretching of the receptor to admit the neurotransmitter molecule has an important function of initiating an energetic stimulation which is missing with the substitute chemical. What the substitute chemical has in its favor is that there are usually more molecules present and they usually provoke a stronger effect than the natural molecule will do.

After stimulating the receiving neuron, the neurotransmitter backs out of the receptor, is free again in the synaptic space, and is drawn to the neuron from which it was originally dispatched. The process can be thought of as docking temporarily before going out to sea again.

The process is very similar to the way the Postal Service operates. The mail person goes to the Post Office, collects your mail, goes out to their truck and drives around town until they come to your home. They deliver your messages or mail but do not stay at your residence. They climb back into their truck, drive back to the Post Office and complete the whole process again the next day.

In the same way, neurotransmitters deliver a chemical message. Then, their job done, they return home to the sending neuron and can either be stored for future use or, if they are aging, can be broken down and replaced. The process then of neurons talking to each other is an electrical, chemical, electrical, and chemical chain of events.

Here is a summary of the chain of actions between neurons:

- A chemical message is received by receptors in the dendrites of a neuron
- It is drawn into the cell body
- An electrical charge is created and moves down the axon
- It reaches the vesicles in the axon terminal nodes
- The vesicles move to the membrane edge
- The vesicles join with the membrane of the neuron and create an opening

- The vesicles release the neurotransmitters into the synapse
- The neurotransmitters go across the gap and plug into the receptors of the receiving neuron
- After stimulating the receiving neuron the neurotransmitters back out of the receptor and go back across the gap
- They are taken back into the sending neuron through re-uptake pumps (called transporters) and can be recycled

Some things can go wrong with this process. When a person takes a substance into their body that is similar to one the body already makes, the body is confused and thinks it is making too much because of the presence of both the neurotransmitter and the outside chemical which mimics it. It may then decide it is working much too hard because of what appears to be an excess of what is needed and may begin to decrease the amount of neurotransmitter it makes. That can progress to the point that the body makes NO neurotransmitter and the person is 'dependent' on taking a chemical in from the outside to supply the missing chemical which the brain/body needs. This process happens in the cell body of the sending neuron.

On the other side of the synapse, the dendrites of the receiving neuron, a couple of things can happen. First, in an effort to protect itself from over- stimulation, some of the receptors can shut down. This is called *Down Regulation*. The opposite effect can also occur in which the dendrites decide there is no way they can handle all the stimulation in the synapse with the limited number of receptors it currently has, and can decide to create more. This then is known as *Up Regulation*. During the process of no longer using an addicting substance the experience will vary depending on whether a person has regulated Up or Down. With *Down Regulation* there is likely to not be enough receptors to adequately stimulate the receiving neuron, and depression or a diminished response may result. When *Up Regulation* has occurred, there may be an increase in craving as the additional receptors are hungry and asking to be fed.

Dependency is really a state in which the body must rely on an outside source for the substituting chemical and then must satisfy the receptors with adequate amounts of the chemical so they do not complain. The discomfort known as withdrawal is basically a combination of the original brain chemical no longer being available, plus the replacement chemical is also missing, and the body reacts by causing symptoms to erupt which draw attention to the fact that it does not feel 'normal' and wants something done about it. The process of recovery then includes an attempt to bring the neuronal processing back to a state of functioning as closely as possible to the original settings, or to improve the original state of affairs which may have played a role in the person's decision to use substances in the first place.

The person in recovery has several options available to them to assist in this process. The intent of this book is not to explore them in detail but only to point to the subject areas that can be explored further if the reader so desires. For some people, community support in the form of Twelve Step groups such as AA/NA/CA or church based activities have been enough. For others, various forms of treatment in a variety of settings aid in the process. This might include residential treatment, intensive outpatient, regular outpatient, Therapeutic Community, detoxification centers, Half-way Houses, etc. Pharmaceutical medications have been designed as an adjunct as well, and have often been prescribed to stabilize the adjustment the body is making to the new 'norm' that is being created.

A more recent and very promising way of addressing the recovery process is using more natural means to re-stabilize the body. This includes attention to the nutritional needs of the body and using supplements in the form of amino acids and co-factors to assist the body in restarting the production process of the neurotransmitters more quickly, as well as significantly decreasing the unpleasant craving. There are several resources for further study which are listed in the bibliography. An increasing number of agencies and therapists in private practice are using these adjuncts with notable success in the prevention of (re)lapsing and the reduction of the initial discomfort in the withdrawal process.

CHAPTER 4

Neurotransmitters

There are somewhere in the neighborhood of one hundred chemicals known as neurotransmitters. Fortunately, we won't be discussing all of them but I have chosen to address the six known to be primary in the use of mind altering chemicals. The information here will be succinct and enough for clinicians or family members who are studying the material to better understand the dilemma of their loved ones. For readers with an interest in more detailed information, there are resources available including some listed in the Bibliography of this text.

The first neurotransmitter we'll discuss is dopamine, an excitatory neurotransmitter. It is designated as such because one of its roles is to help us want to get up in the morning and be interested in participating in life activities. Dopamine is our body's natural cocaine and has several important tasks. It is necessary to help us concentrate and focus. Balancing our checking account, prioritizing the days activities, completing our homework assignments, and planning our vacation all require dopamine. It also is needed to convert an idea we have into physical activity so our body can carry out the suggested activity such as combing your hair, brushing your teeth, taking a drink of water or walking.

The disease that is characteristic of the body's inability to produce adequate dopamine is Parkinson's Disease. People with this unfortunate disorder have ideas but cannot make their body carry them out as the disease progresses. At some point it can even look like they are staring when they are unable to blink their eyes. Dopamine is also a survival neurotransmitter in that the activities needed to keep people here on planet earth release a little dump of dopamine so that they are fun. When we eat we get a little dump of dopamine. When we have sex we get a bigger dump. If eating and having sex weren't fun so we wanted to do them often, people would die out and the species wouldn't survive.

When people use stimulant recreational drugs such as Cocaine, Methamphetamine or Ecstasy, they get a big dump of dopamine, called a 'rush'. They can also experience eating and sex as being rather boring after they discontinue their use of these drugs, since the little sex-dump or food-dump of dopamine is not very impressive in comparison.

GABA is the amino acid that prevents anxiety and fits into the type called inhibitory. It's the body's natural Valium. One way to be suspicious there is not enough GABA is that people have a hard time going to sleep. Their body is tired but their mind won't shut down. You see that with children who have a hard time winding down and going to sleep early. GABA gets dumped into the system following a convulsion or epileptic seizure of some sort. The body has been very stressed during the seizure and needs to have a calming period to reset normal activity. Nature's way of having it relax is to dump in some GABA which then causes the person to be sleepy. It is very common for people to go to sleep following a seizure for this reason. After a fright, GABA is also dumped into the persons system to counteract the effects of the adrenalin rush they have experienced and bring them back to a normal set point for their blood pressure, pulse and respirations.

When people are upset, angry about something, and the situation should now be resolved but they cannot calm down, there may be a deficiency in GABA. Sending a child to their room for a 'time out' if they do not have enough GABA is not an effective disciplinary strategy since they will not calm down. They will yell and scream, bang on the wall, destroy things, and in short, make matters worse. The same thing is true in an adolescent residential treatment facility. When a couple of the youths raise their voices and the staff comes to investigate, they may see them with their 'dukes' up and ready to exchange physical blows. Saying 'time out, off to your rooms' will not be effective either, and they will punch a hole in the wall, tear the drapes down and yell unkind things about the staff. It would be much better to say, 'Come on pal, how about you and I go for a run around the building'. That discharge approach of the chemicals they have released will be more effective than waiting for a GABA dump which might be slow in coming, or unable to come at all.

Research indicates that children who are born into a family with a history of alcohol dependence are often born with low GABA levels and are set up from birth to take in from outside themselves what is missing on the inside. This would mean a likelihood of being drawn to depressants such as alcohol, benzodiazepines or sleeping pills. Anxiety disorders of varying types are also an indicator of GABA problems. Some examples could include problem areas such as panic attacks, phobias, or simply staying in a state of worry about being able to handle life. All drugs in the categories of benzodiazepines, such as Valium, Librium, and Xanax affect the GABA system.

Norepinephrine is made in the body from dopamine and has more specific roles. It is also considered excitatory, and one of its' primary functions is to keep us alert and awake. The highest level most of us have during the day is in the morning, and it is intended to wane as we progress through the day so we can go to sleep at night. We will discuss this further later on, but for now, the difficulty created by eating a heavy protein meal late at night is that this neurotransmitter is activated and it is difficult to go to sleep without the use of alcohol or a sleeping pill.

There are people with very high levels of norepinephrine early in the morning. They awaken without an alarm clock at some early hour, like 4:30am, pop right out of bed, do the vacuuming, put in a couple loads of laundry, sit down at the computer and do a half day's work while everyone else is still in bed. What is also characteristic is that they are often 'finished' with their day at about 3pm, even though they do not go to bed that early, and know not to take on tasks after that time that require attention to detail. There is nothing 'wrong' with their particular rhythm, it is just set to a different internal clock.

Norepinephrine also has a role when we are frightened. When we become aware of a potentially life threatening situation, norepinephrine is activated. It then sends a message to the adrenal gland, located on top of the kidneys, which signals the release of adrenaline (epinephrine) and a whole series of physical changes happen like a domino effect to prepare us to handle the emergency. When people suffer from depression, it may be due to low levels of norepinephrine and they may respond better to antidepressant regimes that influence this neurotransmitter.

Serotonin is another neurotransmitter which is inhibitory. It is our body's natural Prozac or antidepressant. It helps us like ourselves and other people in addition to having a calming emotional effect. Several body functions such as sleeping and eating are affected by serotonin. It is the exact opposite of norepinephrine in that we have none when we wake up in the morning and the body begins to manufacture it, based on the sun cycle. We need a minimum of thirty (30) minutes of sunlight coming into our eyes each day to have enough serotonin to feel good. As the sun begins to go down in the evening, the body stops producing serotonin and converts the serotonin we have into melatonin so we can sleep at night.

When people are deficient in serotonin during the day and struggle with depression, they are also likely to be deficient in melatonin at night and have a corresponding problem with sleeping as well. In locations where the sun is less prominent during the winter time, citizens may have a condition called *Seasonal Affective Disorder* or SAD. They may feel fine during the summer but struggle with depression during the winter months.

There are some easy 'fixes' for these concerns. One is to buy and install full spectrum light bulbs in the home or office. These can be purchased as florescent, halogen or regular lamp bulbs. A more formal Light Box can be purchased, but it is not necessary to go to the additional expense. Chewing increases serotonin levels. When people chew gum a lot, they probably are consciously unaware of the potential improvement in their mood. They just know they like to chew gum. Eating is also a chewing activity and results in gaining weight when people are depressed since they may go to the refrigerator frequently to help with how they are feeling. Just before a women's monthly period, her serotonin level drops and can contribute to the crabbiness associated with PMS.

People who have dominant positions such as managers, CEO's, police officers, fire fighters and gang members often have high serotonin levels. It is much too common that people retire and go home with nothing much planned for their days, and their serotonin levels drop. That may bring on a problem with excessive alcohol use, depression, suicidal thoughts, and an early death. We often have not been successful with rehabilitation of gang members because we tell them to knock off the threatening behaviors but do not help them with alternative activities that boost the feel-good internal chemicals.

The fifth neurotransmitter is endorphin, our natural pain medicine. Like Morphine, it helps us handle both physical and emotional pain. It's what gets dumped into the system when you go jogging. At first you don't feel great, but after about twenty minutes the endorphins kick in and you can run all day. It's the payoff for working out in the gym, and people who do not get much of an endorphin dump generally give up the exercise routine because they don't get a significant reward.

Endorphins help with any kind of emotional pain such as PTSD or domestic violence where there's yelling, name calling, etc. In fact, it's part of the reason people stay in abusive relationships because you don't have to suck your thumb as an adult to self soothe. The endorphins do it for you. When people are low in endorphins they can't self soothe. They over react to things, are emotionally sensitive, and personalize situations. Children who have low levels of endorphins tend to cry a lot and are very sensitive. Their feelings are easily hurt. This is the other neurotransmitter, along with GABA, which research says may be low in children who are born into a family with a history of alcohol dependence.

People with the eating disorder known as Bulimia are often addicted to their own internal endorphins and need assistance with resolving that as well as discontinuing their purging routine. When we vomit, a pain response is often initiated because of the hydrochloric acid and bile back up into the throat area causing a pain reaction that triggers an endorphin dump into the system.

Acetylcholine is the last of the neurotransmitters we will discuss. It has a primary role in activating muscles, both voluntary and involuntary, or those we can control as well as those that work independently of our conscious control. Examples of involuntary muscles might include the iris of the eye which changes the size of the pupil based on the amount of light that is present, and 'growling of the stomach' which we cannot stop even when trying to tighten the abdominal muscles.

Acetylcholine helps maintain moistness throughout the body, regulating the mucous membranes and sweating. In addition, it plays a major role in laying down long term memories in an area of the brain known as the hippocampus. The use of nicotine is the only addicting chemical which first impacts the acetylcholine system. In fact, a deficiency of this neurotransmitter is likely to contribute to beginning the use of tobacco products. After affecting acetylcholine, nicotine then affects all of the other major neurotransmitters which we have discussed. In general, most substance use affects two or three of the major neurotransmitters. Since tobacco use affects all six, it helps to explain why it is so difficult to discontinue its use. In fact, it is common for people in recovery to say that it was easier to discontinue their use of heroin and alcohol than to be successful at discontinuing their nicotine habit.

All of the approximately one hundred neurotransmitters are made from protein. When we eat protein, the body breaks it down to its lowest form which is a series of amino acids. This will be discussed in more detail in Chapter 9, but for now, when we eat protein and it is broken down, the body does this little assay test to see where it is most needed and it will always pick repairing the physical body first. It doesn't really care if you are depressed from not enough serotonin, it wants to keep you alive. So, when there is an inadequate amount of protein, or the body can't make enough of the brain chemicals due to a genetic predisposition, it doesn't allow the brain to have all the chemicals it needs to be balanced and symptoms show up like depression, irritability, tension, anxiety, and craving.

CHAPTER 5

Filling the Vesicles

Several researchers have been interested in how quickly the vesicles are filled. As we discussed earlier, the vesicles are the packets in the nodes of the neurons which contain the neurotransmitters. When I first heard this information, I was fascinated, and as others have continued the study, we now know that there is a pattern which is fairly reliable in terms of chronological age related percentage of filling and the accompanying developmental stages. From the research by Merrill Norton, RPH, University of Georgia, the vesicles are about fifty per cent full by the time a child is eleven years of age, which is why children need parents - they aren't operating on all cylinders yet (my description, not his). By eighteen they are about seventy five per cent full and are not fully matured until the person is twenty-four or twenty-five years of age. This has important implications for the possibility of creating problems in ever reaching maturity.

We know that the use of mind altering chemicals can arrest or interfere with the continuing filling of the vesicles. All of the substances which can be used to alter consciousness mimic at least one of the neurotransmitters. The use of mind altering chemicals would have no effect if the body didn't already make a chemical which did the same thing, except in a much more regulated way and at a much smaller dosage. The reason those substances have the effect they do is that they attach to the receptors intended for the neurotransmitters and create a greatly exaggerated effect in the body.

As discussed in Chapter 3, when an external chemical is taken into the body that mimics a chemical the body makes, the production process of the internal chemicals can be adversely affected. In practical terms, the maturation of an individual can be affected and the full development into functional adulthood may be arrested. Practitioners in the treatment field for substance abuse can attest to the occurrence of clients coming into the program with a chronological age of perhaps thirty-four, but if they began their use of alcohol or marijuana at the age of thirteen their functional development is likely to be still at the thirteen age level. Part of the treatment process should include assisting them in gaining their chronological age so they fit with their age mates in terms of social skills and age related functioning.

CHAPTER 6

Some Hereditary Factors

The more people in the family line with alcohol dependence, the more likely it is that the children will be predisposed to drinking. There is some research to indicate that the stronger the history, the earlier the children are likely to choose some external substance to soothe themselves. Even when alcohol is not used by the child, they often pick other things such as sugar. Sugar is usually the first addiction for most people, and some researchers go so far as to say it IS the first addiction.

The research of Dr. Norton is particularly helpful in understanding the role of a family history of dependence and its impact on the possible development of the children's pattern of alcohol use. He divides the types of people who begin to use heavily into three separate categories. The first is the Environmental Alcoholic. This is a person with no family history of alcohol use, significant mental health issues, suicides or significant trauma. When this young person goes on a 'kegger' with friends in the tenth grade he (or she) will think that was interesting, even fun, but won't be driven to repeat the experience often.

However, when he goes to college and begins a style of drinking on the weekends with buddies, this behavior may be continued following graduation. In that situation, his neurotransmitter loads may never reach one hundred percent and he may begin to experience difficulty in maintaining an active and energetic lifestyle in mid-life. He may come home at the end of a day feeling drained and not have the energy to participate in family activities. Most often there isn't a problem with performance evaluations at work or frequent calling in with the 'flu', but the energy level after the day's work is dragging.

He most likely will see his physician and after describing his situation, which can easily be diagnosed as depression, he likely will go home with a prescription for an antidepressant without ever really sharing about the drinking pattern. Because of a more robust genetic predisposition, he may be able to drink heavily for fifteen to twenty years with minimal issues. This type of alcoholic might be called a *functional alcoholic* because they don't draw attention to themselves and their drinking. Family members, friends or employers aren't particularly concerned about their drinking; it is more an internal loss of personal vitality that the person experiences.

The second pattern is called Type 1 Alcoholic-Adult Onset. This child will have a family history either down the male or female side and it can be passed on either to males or females. This child may go on a 'kegger' in the tenth grade and the response will be very different. The conclusion will be that this is 'good stuff'. They immediately feel exhilarated and will report that they can think better and feel more 'normal', the way they perceive how others feel when not under the influence. In the past when they reported that they could think or perform better, they were often told it was 'a bunch of bull'; however there is some truth to what they are saying.

A family history of dependence on alcohol may mean that the child is born with the potential for lower levels of neurotransmitter production and this child may level out at about 60%. Their experience will then mean that when they drink, it dumps more neurotransmitters into the synapse than is usually available and the result would be increased availability for sending messages more efficiently to neighboring neurons. If we remember the pattern and rate of filling the vesicles with neurotransmitters, this makes sense.

Since they have such a wonderful experience, they will want to repeat the 'drinking to get drunk' pattern often and they likely will begin in their High School years drinking heavily and regularly to get the exhilaration. It also may mean that there will be a shorter drinking career of twelve to fifteen years before they come to someone's attention. Many people with dual problem areas in their lives of both alcohol abuse and distressing mental health symptoms fall into this category. The use of alcohol becomes a way of managing their lives while at the same time creating further issues. This is a population that may be plagued with lapse issues unless something is done to assist both with the craving patterns and the ability of the body to produce the neurotransmitters in sufficient amounts to stabilize and normalize their brain functioning.

The third group is referred to as Alcoholic Type II – Adolescent Onset. This research focused on the impact down the male side of the family; however, we are seeing more girls now who seem to be following a similar pattern. This will be a child born with very low neurotransmitter load potential which may be as low as ten to twenty five percent. Their very first use of alcohol will result in a dramatic effect, so much so that they are likely to begin drinking heavily at a very early age. My own clinical experience has included awareness of a person that had his first drunk at six years of age and began 'drinking to get drunk' very often, which led to problem use being expressed very early in life. This type of alcoholic predisposition can result in becoming a 'full blown' alcoholic in two years and can resemble a much older person in terms of the withdrawal process. Because their neurotransmitters are so low, they struggle with learning and developing appropriate relationships with family members as well as peers. While I was Director of a residential program, which included responsibility for the adolescent unit, looking at the school work of many of the adolescents confirmed that they were functioning at a second or third grade level.

When they drink excessively, more neurotransmitters than usual are released into the synapse which they experience as a significant shift in their processing and functioning ability. They then 'fall in love' with alcohol, using it often and heavily. As a result of their early and heavy use, they begin to experience physical decline and can develop serious conditions, including death, at an early age. They characteristically do not appear intoxicated even after a Blood Alcohol Level (BAL) test confirms that they are indeed drunk. They can maintain a very high BAL, maybe in the .5 or above range and appear to functioning quite well. They aren't staggering about, bumping into things, they remember their phone number and address, and can appear quite lucid. Their friends may remark that they can 'drink others under the table' or 'hold their liquor' and both the person and their friends may consider this a blessing, thinking that they just have a better constitution than others. In fact, they are at greater risk of physical complications and death at an earlier age due to their inherent weaknesses and their early and heavy use of alcohol.

This information from Dr. Norton is a gift in understanding and registering what may be contributing to the using pattern of clients, friends, and loved ones. Many students in my classes have reported that they easily identify clients they have worked with, and the pattern is clear now in terms of the differences in their use and physical decline. The information is also useful as a guide in the treatment process, understanding the potential for mental health concerns as well as lapse patterns.

CHAPTER 7

The Brain

The brain is a marvelous organ weighing about three pounds and containing about one hundred billion neurons. In the later months in the fetal development process the cortex or outer rim begins folding in on itself to make room for more neurons so that at the time of birth it looks like a gnarled walnut. That provides the fetus with the ability to learn anything that it wants to and as the stimulation and learning process proceeds, the cortex shapes itself according to use. Neurons that aren't asked to do anything decide they aren't needed and begin to prune away. It is said that the brain is the only organ in the entire body that doesn't need to get old. It can continually change itself according to use and stimulation. That knowledge has helped to change our care for elders by providing book clubs, sing a-longs and pottery classes in the facilities that care for them and helping them to remain vital in their mental abilities.

For our purposes, learning the names of all the components of the brain isn't necessary, however, the basic areas and their primary function is useful information to understand.

If we review the brain structure, beginning at its base is the brain stem, also referred to as the Reptilian Brain. It sits on top of the spinal cord. It is called the Reptilian Brain because we share it in common with reptiles and it is the only brain component that reptiles have. It is responsible to keep them alive. As such, it regulates blood pressure, heart rate, breathing, mating, hunger and thirst. They live entirely by instinct, mating when an internal signal suggests it's time to find a partner and lay eggs for future generations, and eating when they are hungry.

It also provides a mechanism for protection when they are threatened. It's called 'freezing'. They take a big gulp of air and go to the bottom of the swamp or pond. This automatically resets their brain to slow the heart rate so less oxygen is needed and they can remain under water for a longer period of time than usual. When they think the danger may be gone, they come up to check and either get another gulp of air and return to the bottom or continue with their life functions with no further concern about a threat.

There is a corresponding function in humans. This part of our brain keeps our body alive by regulating the same functions as a crocodile. One difference is the freezing response. Humans cannot 'freeze' at the same level as reptiles or they would die, however, there can be a partial freeze which might be labeled as depression. When the reptilian brain is affected in a negative way, for instance by substances of abuse, there is a possibility that the risk of death is increased. For instance, this can happen when a young person decides to demonstrate that now they are a mature adult when they celebrate their twenty first birthday by drinking twenty one drinks of alcohol as fast as they can. As the brain tissue becomes saturated it will reach the brain stem, and since alcohol is a sedative, it will 'put it to sleep'. We call this *alcohol poisoning*. Their friends may simply say they will let the person 'sleep it off' with an often unfortunate result of not waking up again. Essentially all the energetic signals needed to keep the body alive and functioning have been dampened and the respective organs fail to function. This obviously has happened too many times on college campuses where excessive drinking has, unfortunately, become part of the college experience. In addition, this part of the brain is 'reset' when a user of chemical substances crosses from an abuse status to dependency.

The emotional brain, called the Limbic System (and also referred to as the Mammalian Brain), sits above the brain stem and is responsible for launching all emotional states. When a person has difficulty expressing emotions, we might wonder about the health of this part of the brain. Both GABA and Serotonin have a role here in maintaining emotional stability. Antidepressants and Benzodiazepines work by affecting this part of the brain. They reduce worry and depressive feelings, allowing the sense of self to be at peace so emotional balance or states of sleep can easily occur.

We share this part of the brain with all mammals whose limbic brain allows them to have some capacity for emotional bonding. As an example, your dog wags its tail when you arrive home after the day's work and is happy to see you. Horses have a relationship with their owner. Animals are known for their ability to detect when humans or other animals are sick and to tend to them in a caring way.

This part of the brain is larger in women than men, which helps to explain two things; women are more prone to depression than men, and there is no culture in the world where men are the primary caregivers of children. There certainly are some 'stay at home dads' who assume the major role in the daily care of children, however, that is not the usual pattern. When this part of the brain is impacted by the use of addicting chemicals, there is a corresponding affect on the stability of emotional states. This might also be exaggerated because another part of the brain, the prefrontal cortex (PFC), has been numbed so the user feels freer to follow any urges they might have without the oversight of the PFC to say 'no'. The Limbic System is in the maturing phase during adolescence so the behavior of people who use substances often mimics the adolescent period of development.

The outer rim of the brain is called the Cortex and is responsible for many functions such as sensory perception and interpretation, thinking, problem solving, and concentration. The part we're most interested in is just behind the forehead and is called the Prefrontal Cortex. It is the 'thinking brain' and helps in tasks such as balancing the bank statement, completing homework assignments and processing information. Dopamine is the dominant neurotransmitter here and enables the person to make decisions that are in their best interest. It has oversight responsibility and one of its primary functions is to inhibit emotional responses when appropriate. It functions as the parent who acknowledges that an impulse seems like a fun thing to do but doesn't allow the behavior because it might not turn out well or be safe.

It's obvious that when this part of the brain is hampered in some way, especially from the use of substances, that the parental function has been impaired and the person may participate in activities that might be dangerous, say things they will regret later, or make decisions that can impact their life later on. An example might be choosing to buy more Crack rather than paying the rent.

Surrounding the brain, and just inside the skull, is a protective mechanism called the Blood Brain Barrier (BBB). It is composed of several membranes and a capillary system which is connected to larger blood vessels which lie on top of the BBB. The purpose of the BBB is to protect the brain from being exposed to situations it shouldn't need to deal with and to provide a bit of a cushion which minimizes bruising and damage to the brain tissue from falls or bumps.

One way it protects the brain is to allow only fat soluble things to cross over into the brain. Since most addicting substances are fat soluble they readily gain access and then create the drug experience that the user wants. When substances are water soluble they are prevented from crossing in most cases. There are some exceptions such as cocaine which is water soluble and has another mechanism for crossing into the brain. Pharmaceutical drugs can be created in such a way that they either readily cross, if the brain needs to be involved, or they are prevented from crossing and remain in the larger blood vessel system.

As substances are taken into the body they are taken up into the circulatory system. When they enter the vessels which lie on top of the brain, and if they are fat soluble, they may be easily taken into the brain. Their first impact will be on what lies closest to the outer rim. Since that is where the sensation and thinking areas are located, the response will be a numbing of those functions. As a result, people often feel exhilaration since their social appropriateness learning will have been dampened. It is common for people to laugh more, even at things that aren't really very funny, and to begin to participate in activities that might more nearly resemble adolescent behavior.

Once inside the brain the substance can begin a chain reaction from one component of the brain to another, which can result in stimulating the Pleasure Pathway, or begin a slowing of function. The Pleasure Pathway is named for the cascade movement of stimulation from one part of the brain to others, resulting in a satisfying and usually stimulating experience. As greater amounts of the substance are introduced into the brain, the tissues on the surface become saturated and the underlying tissues are then affected. So, in domino fashion, the thinking brain is affected, then the emotional brain, and if the substance continues to be taken in, the brain stem and physical safety will be influenced.

Since we know that the brain controls body function, there can be a corresponding impact on body organs and functioning. Not only is the brain sending messages to body organs, but they may be suffering from the direct effect of the substance traveling through the circulatory system reaching them as well. There then can be more immediate effects such as the drug high or intoxication symptoms, or after frequent or prolonged use, the effects can be longer lasting, and in some cases, contribute to the ultimate death of the person.

So, what are we to do? Clearly removing the toxins is the first step. That is, stopping the progression of a behavior that has created chaos and havoc in the person's life. As we march through history there have been a variety of interventions, some helpful, some not, some silly, some unethical. As mentioned in Chapter 3, the primary focus in more recent history has been 'talk therapy' ranging from visits to a pastor or priest, Twelve Step groups such as AA, CA, and NA and including more formal treatment programs. The statistics about outcome are varied and discouraging for the most part.

There began to be some curious seekers who wondered about the role of going back to how the body was created, what it needs in order to thrive, and the miracle that is experienced every day as the body automatically repairs itself. Just perhaps, an additional approach of assisting the body in that effort through more natural means, the ones it is *used* to, might make a difference in the success of people who are asking for and needing some assistance in changing their lifestyle into a more successful and healthier mode!

CHAPTER 8

Does Nutrition Have a Role in Recovery?

One of the most exciting things we are learning is that there is a reason that people begin using a substance. They are not just weak willed, lacking in character or being a jerk. They are *using* to change the way they feel due to a brain and body that is out of balance. That also means we can identify children at risk as we watch their behavior and do something about it before they begin having problems with using, problems with relationships, or problems feeling good about themselves. So, the next question is what to do.

The field of substance abuse treatment has adopted the stance that addiction has a bio-psycho-social etiology, but many agencies have used a psycho-social model only in the treatment regime. There is a plethora of research documents which demonstrate convincingly that addressing the biological component is essential in stabilizing recovery. A major factor contributing to the absence of a nutritional/biological component in treatment is the lack of awareness in the medical and clinical communities of the value of addressing these factors. Most clinicians will confirm that a client in the group or individual treatment setting who is 'white knuckling' it and wishing desperately for a drink is not profiting from the treatment process at that time. Another factor is the reluctance of agencies and treatment providers to change their internal system to include a new approach. When the Policies and Procedures are all written and the staff is trained, it is easier to continue with the protocol in place.

It is not useful to be critical of what has happened in the past but to look forward to moving the treatment field along with the implementation of the additional information we have available. Some programs use a sophisticated supplementation process of amino acids and co-factors and their clinical outcomes are extraordinary. The intent of this text is not to address these options in detail but to suggest that readers explore the references in the bibliography to enhance their knowledge base.

Instead, I am going to address a more simplistic approach which is to integrate accurate nutritional information with the hope that changing the basic way we feed clients, and the information we give them about how they can influence their own healing and recovery process throughout their life, will make a major impact on the success rates of the recovery field.

The information about what and how we should eat is both confusing and maddening. It is often contradictory and books are written espousing a variety of dramatically different ways of feeding the human body. It is likely that I will add to the mix in the information I want to share, but I ask the reader to explore for themselves the validity rather than taking the traditional information as truth. The intent here is not to address eating patterns for weight reduction or to compare various diets for effectiveness. Instead, I want to focus on the role of nutrients in the body and then address some nutritional guidelines for people in early recovery.

I acknowledge that agencies often do the best they can with limited resources; however, it is also troubling that sometimes they aren't open to the changes that would be required when information suggests more effective ways of serving their clients. For instance, food banks can be a source of foodstuffs which are less expensive. However, there is a temptation to bring back into the facility some things, because they are cheap, that are not nutritious or in the best interest of the clients. Day old products are also available from grocery stores but often include donuts, bagels, and other pastries. As we will discuss, one problem with this method of feeding clients includes using these foods as the breakfast menu and begins the day on empty carbohydrates which set the client up to be both drowsy and hungry again very quickly.

The timing of the nutrients that are consumed contributes either to alertness or drowsiness. In general, proteins are 'wakeup' foods and provide the nutrients needed to make the neurotransmitters. The guideline for the expected effect from food is as follows: in one (1) hour the full effect will be in place which will last for four (4) hours. It begins to wane in the fifth hour. As a result, when a dietary regime is followed where the highest percentage of protein consumed during the day is taken late in the evening, people will experience difficulty going to sleep without the aid of some alcohol or a sleeping pill. For clients in recovery, as well as people in general, the meal with the highest amount of protein should be consumed at breakfast, followed by lunch, and the lightest protein should be reserved for the evening meal. This will enable the brain to think, focus, process information, complete homework assignments, as well as stay alert with a healthy sense of self in relationship with other people.

Carbohydrates on the other hand are defocusing or 'go to sleep' foods, especially simple carbohydrates. When the day is begun with a bowl of cereal, pancakes, waffles, bagels, orange juice and a banana they all send a message about 'chilling out' and the usual routine is to stop for a coffee drink on the way to work to offset the 'go to sleep' message from the breakfast. This type of breakfast fed to clients in a residential setting will ensure that when they come to group, unless they stop and get a can of a stimulant drink from the pop machine on the way, they will struggle with being sleepy. The reverse is true in the evening. Because they have had significant protein late in the day when the staff wishes them to be in bed so they can attend to the charting and chores that need their attention, the clients are having trouble going to sleep, are up wandering about, wanting to talk until late into the evening. Simply adjusting the timing of the types of foods introduced throughout the day can have a significant impact on the ability to participate fully as well as treatment outcomes.

There are three basic food groups; protein, fat, and carbohydrates. They each have a role in creating and maintaining a healthy, well functioning body and nervous system.

CHAPTER 9

Protein

As we discussed earlier in Chapter 4, all of the approximately one hundred neurotransmitters are made in the body from the protein that we eat. Protein can't be used by the body in the form we take it in. It has to be broken down into the basic molecules which are called amino acids. It is commonly accepted that there are twenty two (22) of these, and they are divided into groups called essential and non-essential. In a way, this is a misnomer because it is easy to misunderstand and think that it is necessary to have the essential ones, and the others are nice but not necessary. What the words really mean is that it is necessary to eat the essential ones in the daily diet, and if these are present, the body can then make the others internally.

The amino acids are like little pop beads that can be joined together in a number of different ways to complete a variety of tasks. For instance, they can be joined together to make testosterone, dopamine or thyroxin, as well as muscle and body tissue. The primary concern of the amino acids is to keep the body alive, so the priority is always to repair body tissue rather than making chemicals that keep us happy and enjoying life. For instance, if you work out in the gym and your muscles are sore, the body repairs those muscles first, and then makes things like Serotonin. It follows then that an inadequate amount of protein or protein of inferior quality can result in deficiencies of the chemicals needed to maintain a high quality of life.

There are two types of protein, complete and incomplete. The complete proteins have all nine of the essential amino acids, and the body can then make the nonessential ones to provide for all the body functions which are dependent on the tasks that protein provides. Meat products, especially fatty fish, are the best sources of complete proteins, with the plant forms being the incomplete family of proteins. A plant form may have four of the essential amino acids and must be combined with another plant at the same time which has the other five. An example might be the combination of unprocessed forms of rice and beans. When they are eaten at the same time the body is able to complete the process of building the nonessential ones and continue to support all of the life processes dependent on amino acids. People who have chosen a lifestyle as a vegetarian or vegan can be very healthy; however, the challenge for them will be ensuring that all of the essential amino acids are available in their diet. This usually necessitates careful planning. Every now and then there is 'news' that a plant protein is complete. In general, that information is later followed with 'news' that it isn't. Some examples have been soy and spirulina.

There is a well documented list of tasks that amino acids perform, including stabilizing blood sugar, preventing seizures, inhibiting the growth of the herpes virus, and aiding in blood clotting in addition to the production of neurotransmitters. So it becomes apparent that deficiencies can lead to many situations in the body that result in imbalance and the appearance of physical symptoms. A potential concern about using protein 'Bars' is that the number of grams does not ensure that the essential ones are all present.

On the other hand, moderation is also important. The body can only process a small amount at a time and the excess is converted to fat and stored on various parts of the body. Another issue with excessive use is the effect on the body's pH since proteins, especially meats, are acidic and the body functions better in a slightly alkaline state. Fruits and vegetables are alkaline in nature and help to achieve this balance.

CHAPTER 10

Fats

This family of nutrients has been misrepresented in our culture starting back as early as the years following World War II. We were told that butter and lard weren't good for us and some plastics were made as replacements, namely margarine and shortening. In fact, the early margarine was white and came in a plastic bag with a capsule of food coloring that you opened and then mixed together to resemble the color of butter.

In my own study of researchers in the field, I now am firmly of the opinion that as a country we have suffered devastating physical issues as a result. Since the intent of this discussion is not to defend the use of saturated fats, (there are resources in the Bibliography), I will only address how the use/misuse of fats affects the nervous system and can impact the efficient functioning of the brain and all nervous tissue. That is important because if there is to be successful healing in the substance abuse field, attention must be paid to repairing brain tissue and function.

The myelin sheath is in part made from saturated fat which provides structure and stability to the neuron. In addition, it creates a healthy membrane over which electrolytes like sodium and potassium can move. When they move back and forth across the membrane an electrical charge is created which then moves down the axon and stimulates the release of the neurotransmitters into the synaptic gap. When the myelin is not well-formed, it interferes with the electrical current in the nervous system. Moderation is the guideline here but there are so many more ways in which a fat free diet or missing saturated fat in the diet can lead to significant health issues.

There are four types of fat. The saturated group gets its name because there is a carbon chain of varying lengths and each of the carbons has a hydrogen molecule attached to it - hence the name 'saturated'. The number of carbons can vary and are referred to as a short, medium or long chain fat and the chains lie in a straight line. Butter, lard, coconut oil and palm oil are all examples of saturated fats.

They can all be used in cooking since they are stable and do not become rancid (explained later). There are many tasks of saturated fat in the body, such as making fatty pads on the hands, feet, and under the seat bones (which you want to have if you ride horses). It also escorts calcium into the bones to prevent bone disease and provides satiation so you aren't tempted to overeat. It helps to make healthy myelin sheaths as part of the neuron. Numerous other benefits teach us that we need some if we are to be as healthy as possible.

Monounsaturated fats have a missing hydrogen, because two carbons snuggle up to each other and share a single hydrogen. This is called a double bond, and at that point in the chain it bends just a little so the chain now begins to go upwards a bit. Olive oil is an example here and can be used in cooking without concern about rancidity either.

Polyunsaturated fats have many double bonds and so the chain is no longer straight or has a slight bend. It can look more like a backwards letter C. There are several types, but I will mention only two here. A general rule is that these oils should not be used in cooking because they form a polymer, a plastic, which interferes with digestion. An example would be corn oil which is an Omega-6 fat. It is inflammatory to cell walls and when heated becomes rancid and throws off free radicals which are damaging to body tissue. Most 'vegetable' oils fit into this category.

Free radicals are oxygen components that have broken away from their home molecule, are oxidized (rust), and go exploring their world. At some point they are tired of being alone and want to find another family so start banging into cells asking for acceptance and causing little dents known as free radical damage. Free radical damage is a natural part of the aging process; however, lifestyle issues and substance use contributes to the intensity of the damage.

Another one of these fats is Omega-3 and is found in fatty fish like salmon and flaxseed oil. Omega-3 is considered to be 'brain food' and is necessary for the health of the myelin sheath. A study at Harvard determined that Bipolar Disorder could be greatly improved by using salmon oil capsules. There is increasing evidence to confirm that Omega-3 has an important role in brain health and repair from the use of toxins.

The last fat I'll mention is Trans fat which means going across, like Trans Atlantic flights which cross the ocean. In this situation, a catalyst like Nickel is used to cause the hydrogen molecules to jump across the chain with the result that two hydrogen molecules are attached to one carbon on one side of the chain. If all the hydrogen molecules jump across, the fat is hydrogenated. If only some of them go across, it is a partially hydrogenated fat.

Recent concerns have prompted government officials to make new rulings about the use of trans fat since they have been shown to be very detrimental to the human body. Many products now say on the front of the packaging that there is 'No Trans Fat'. However, if you look at the ingredient list you notice either hydrogenated or partially hydrogenated oils. The new ruling is that if a product contains no more than .5 gram of Trans fat per serving in the container it can be listed as 'No Trans Fat'. Trans fats look like saturated fat to the cell membrane and it allows it to enter, then creates havoc because it cannot be used in any of the functions of a saturated fat and essentially plugs up the cell.

Encouraging clients to eat fats which assist in the repair process will speed along their success in recovery and facilitate a high quality of brain health and balance. The best fats for this purpose are saturated fats, monounsaturated and Omega -3. A saturated fat that is particularly healing is coconut oil - especially for people with liver disease. It does not tax the liver by requiring bile to be produced by the liver to break it down for use in the digestive tract, so its use provides a rest period allowing the liver to better heal itself.

CHAPTER 11

Carbohydrates

Carbohydrates can be divided into two primary groups: simple and complex. Those words simply refer to the speed with which they are converted into a sugar (glucose) in the body. That is an important issue because when the process happens quickly, there is a corresponding spike in blood sugar and the body responds by dumping several things into the system, such as insulin and cortisol.

The molecules of alcohol and glucose are almost identical. Alcohol is fermented sugar, and people with a predisposition to alcohol abuse, or in recovery, need to be cautious about simple carbohydrates that break down very quickly into sugar in the blood stream. When that happens, it sets up a craving for more sugar and alcohol. Foods like fruit juice, white bread, and pasta can be problematic. It's much better to eat the fruit itself rather than simply drinking the juice because the body has to work at getting the sugar out. The glucose blood level then rises more slowly, avoiding an insulin and cortisol dump which can set people up for problems such as diabetes or adrenal exhaustion.

It takes about three days to detoxify from a sugar addiction and even though the person will experience some craving, it is not problematic like alcohol detoxification which can have life threatening problems. Craving is the worst feature and if people endure that for the three days, the craving goes away but will quickly return if simple sugars are reintroduced into the diet, especially in large quantities.

Even though carbohydrates are not necessary for building or maintaining the structure of the neuron or the production of the chemicals which allow them to talk to each other, they have an important role in providing fuel for body functions and maintaining a healthy pH balance. Another important intended function of carbohydrates is the supplying of vitamins, minerals and enzymes the body needs. Unfortunately, the majority of foods produced for consumption today have been altered in their chemical makeup which is called hybridization.

Since we like out-of-season foods which are not produced nearby all year round, we import foods from far away. This means they need to be prepared to withstand the journey, storage in warehouses, being moved about in large vans, and ultimately ending up on the shelf in the super market. A naturally grown fruit would have ripened and begun to decay or rot by the time this arduous journey was completed and would not be acceptable either to the grocer or to the customers who would turn up their noses at the sight of them. In order to avoid this unhappy outcome, researchers have learned how to hybridize or change the chemical makeup of the fruit or vegetable so there would be a longer shelf life. This is accomplished by removing some of the enzymes from the item which are intended to help us digest them when they are taken into the intestinal tract. Obviously their nutritional value has been reduced.

In addition, the soil in which many of these products are grown has been over used, planting the same crop repeatedly which removes essential components from the soil. The resultant product does not have the vitamins and minerals that nature intended we should get from them, making the use of supplements of vitamins and minerals necessary. Clearly the use of pesticides, fertilizers, coloring agents and preservatives has added to this problem.

If we go back to the issue of substance abuse and the impact of nutrition, amino acids by themselves aren't enough to produce a healthy batch of neurotransmitters. The vitamins and minerals are referred to as co-factors and are necessary ingredients in the production process. If we think of the cells in the body as each being a factory with the job of producing a product of some sort and there is a railroad track going by with train cars bringing in the coal and raw materials, it is very similar to the cells with a nearby blood vessel system bringing in all the nutrients.

We could use the analogy of deciding we want to make a chocolate cake, which isn't the best for our discussion but apt nonetheless. So we begin to gather all the ingredients. We get out the eggs, flour, sugar, and cocoa and then discover we are out of baking powder. We might say 'oh darn' and then decide to make the cake anyway. As we are mixing it, and putting it in the pan and the oven it looks like a chocolate cake. However, when we take it out of the oven it will look more like brownies. In a similar way, when important ingredients are missing when a batch of dopamine is being mixed, the outcome will be a defective batch. The co-factors include things such as iron, Vitamin C, various B Vitamins, and copper. They should all be readily available and easily obtained through our diet, and the fruits and vegetables we eat are nature's way of obtaining these nutrients.

There is a ladder-like process of making the neurotransmitters. As one step is completed, additional co-factors are needed to move to the next step. In this way there is a conversion of the basic amino acid into the neurotransmitters like serotonin or dopamine. So, in a very real way, what we eat and the quality of the food we eat matters in our health and vitality. Sometimes people fear that eating more organic foods will be more costly. Often though, they discover that eating better will result in eating less as the body will be satisfied instead of asking for more since it can't find what it needs.

CHAPTER 12

Water

The role of water must be included in a discussion about brain chemistry and the role of nutrition in recovery. Approximately 75% of the body is water which is distributed between the inside of the cells, forming an ocean for the cells to swim in, and in the blood. The ratio is approximately 66% in the cells, 26% in the fluid surrounding the cells, and 8% in the blood volume. Dehydration is one of the most difficult problems for the body to handle and creates a stress reaction that is manifested in various organs as they struggle to cope. As F. Batmanghelidj, MD states in his book, *You're Not Sick, You're Thirsty*, 'When a new dehydration-produced chemical state becomes fully established, it causes many structural changes, even to the genetic blueprints of the body'.

Water regulates all body functions. It has a hydraulic function created by little turbine like pumps on the cell membrane which force potassium into the cell and push sodium out. Water generates the energy to turn the pumps by becoming sticky at the cell wall. Sodium and potassium stick to the pump and when the pump turns quickly it creates an electrical charge which energizes the cell.

Water is the adhesive that binds solid parts of the cell together and provides the best 'pick me up' when we need more energy. If there is not enough water to adequately provide this energy function we will need to rely on food. If there is a deficit, the body sets up a reserve plan very much like the city guidelines for water use during a drought. The city leaders ask that you shower rather than taking a tub bath, don't flush the stool each time it is used, and water the lawn for only fifteen minutes before 10am or after 6pm on alternating days. In addition, the distribution of the water into the city is restricted through decreasing the amount released from the reservoirs, and sometimes setting up additional reservoirs.

Drought in the body causes distress of body systems. To begin our understanding of how this works, we'll start with the roles of the kidneys and salt. Water and salt need to be balanced and it is the kidneys' job to regulate fluid by either releasing or preventing the loss of salt from the body. The point is not to prevent any salt intake. We need the Sodium component to cross over the membranes with Potassium to make energy. We need the Chloride molecule to make hydrochloric acid in the stomach to help with food digestion. Moderation is again the guiding principle. In dehydration salt is not allowed to be released from the kidneys in an attempt to retain water in the body. Reservoirs are temporarily created to hold the fluid that is absolutely required for the major organs to function and maintain life. Edema is the result and may be noticed in soft tissue such as around the ankles.

Other changes are made as well in the reserve plan, one of which is in the respiratory system. Each time we exhale we lose water from the lungs. If you put a mirror under your nose and exhale onto it tiny beads of moisture will collect. In drought, the bronchiole tubes which escort air in and out of the lungs constrict and reduce the size of their opening in an effort to reduce water loss. Wheezing from an asthma attack can be due to restricted tubules through which to breathe. Thickened phlegm is another indicator. The fluid from the membranes should be watery in nature.

The digestive tract needs water to process food. It has some priority and will take water from other body functions to provide saliva. We will not have a dry mouth until the deficit is severe. The stomach has a row of cells on the lining which make sodium bicarbonate ($NaCO_3$). The bicarbonate neutralizes the hydrochloric acid (HCL) produced in the stomach and protects the stomach wall from acid damage. There must be water to make bicarbonate and the result of not enough water to perform this function is heartburn.

Another important role of water in the digestive system is to protect the small intestines by making bicarbonate in the pancreas. When food is eaten it cannot leave the stomach until it is liquid. Then a signal goes to a round muscle called a sphincter that looks like a donut with a hole in the middle. This is the connecting place between the stomach and the small intestines. In order to dump the stomachs contents both the stomach and the small intestines must signal that they are ready. The stomach initiates this signal saying, in effect, 'I've done my part, everything is in liquid form'. Then the small intestine needs to reply saying it is either ready or not for company. If there is plenty of water the pancreas will have done its job of making some more bicarbonate so it can neutralize the acidic mixture as it arrives.

The signal from the underneath side of the sphincter won't allow food to dump into the small intestine unless there is enough bicarbonate to neutralize the acid as it comes through the sphincter. The lining of the intestines is different from the lining of the stomach and would be permanently damaged if the acidic contents were dumped in with no ability to neutralize it. If bicarbonate is not available the underside of the sphincter says 'no way' and does not allow the dump, which creates a situation in which the person will still feel full, many hours after eating. There are only two ways to exit the stomach and if the door to the intestines is blocked, people may have the urge to vomit as the only other alternative.

When we drink water, a hormone/neurotransmitter called *motilin* is secreted which produces peristalsis, the muscular movement causing the liquid food to move through the intestinal tract. All the nutrients from food are extracted here and absorbed into the circulatory system for distribution to body cells. The production of brain chemicals (neurotransmitters) is dependent on the gastrointestinal tract working well.

There are other significant organ symptoms that indicate distress from draught, and if the reader is curious to learn more, I heartily suggest the works of Dr. Batmanghelidj listed in the Bibliography. We won't be addressing those here as the focus is on brain function and the role of nutrition.

In brief, if medication is used to deal with the distress it will silence the signal but will not cure the problem. Dehydration eventually causes loss of some functions and produces damage (pathology).

So the question is 'How much water do we need?' Every twenty four hours the body recycles available water to maintain normal physiological functions resulting in a shortage of about six to ten glasses of water each day. It has to be replaced every day and must be 'free' water with no chemicals that the liver has to process. A useful guideline to follow is: half the body weight in ounces. So if a person weighs one hundred sixty pounds, eighty ounces of water should be the goal. In addition, caffeine is very drying because it signals the kidney to work harder and more urine is produced. People who drink coffee in the morning can attest to this as they will need to release this buildup soon after drinking. To offset this additional drying affect, three more containers of water the size of the coffee or caffeine container needs to be added to the daily requirement.

Water intake should be spaced out during the day to maximize the benefits. Drinking some water about thirty minutes before meals and more about two hours after meals helps prepare both the stomach and the intestines for the food that will soon be coming. It is better not to drink a lot of water with meals because this dilutes the digestive enzymes. However, if that's all the water a person is drinking, they should 'go for it'.

CHAPTER 13

Eating For Recovery

How can all this information be helpful as people are struggling with their recovery process? First of all, a balanced diet using nutritious foods is a starting place. Then there are some specific suggestions for what to eat and what to avoid especially in early recovery. I will outline some of these suggestions with the hope that they will be tools not only for people in recovery and their loved ones, but also for practitioners in the health care fields. Since the use of toxins affects different neurotransmitters, there are some substance related suggestions for consideration.

Because alcohol and glucose are almost identical, the use of simple sugars for persons in recovery from that substance should be avoided. That would include things like white bread and rice, most pastas, potatoes, and sugar products. It is also better to eat the fruit rather than fruit juice because the body has to work harder at releasing the juice from the fruit, preventing a spike in the blood sugar resulting in craving.

People can blow a BAL of .02 due only to their pattern of eating, called an 'auto brewery effect'. For instance, eating a banana at the same time as a heavy meat product means the banana will be in liquid form in the stomach in a short period of time, about twenty minutes, but it has to sit and wait, twiddling it's thumbs so to speak, until the meat is also in liquid form before the stomach will dump the contents into the small intestine. Depending on the meat product eaten, that can take quite awhile. In the meantime, it is moist and warm in the stomach and fermentation can occur. The BAL level is enough to set up craving for alcohol from an outside source. A useful guideline here is to use fruits as a snack between meals or as a dessert.

When people are healing from the use of heroin or pharmaceutical narcotics there are two foods groups that can be problematic: grains and dairy. The reason is that the stomach can make two narcotic-like substances, gluteomorphin and caseomorphin. Those substances can obviously create an internal stimulation which initiates craving and interferes with the commitment to stay clean. They also have a dulling or dampening effect like heroin, which is why we call them 'comfort foods'.

Because chocolate attaches to the same receptors as marijuana, it is common for people to begin a heavy use of chocolate while trying to discontinue their use of marijuana. People have been known to gain an additional thirty pounds after stopping the use of the drug because of using milk chocolate products. Using seventy or eighty per-cent dark chocolate products instead helps prevent this problem. There is some information that dark chocolate has some healthful components and that using nibs, dried cacao beans, in cooking and food products, adds some useful elements while avoiding the blood sugar spike.

Both methamphetamine and cocaine users can benefit from high quality protein, especially early in the day. That allows the raw materials to be available to make dopamine and norepinephrine, the excitatory neurotransmitters they have affected by their drug use.

For tobacco users, acetylcholine is made from lecithin in our foods. Lecithin is found in things such as egg yolks, liver, fatty fish, wheat germ, organic peanut butter, beef, hazelnuts, macadamia nuts, and soy protein powder.

CHAPTER 14

Supplements

The basic reason to use supplements such as amino acids and co-factors in treating persons with substance related concerns is that they jump start the brain into reversing the production shut down of the neurotransmitters. That also makes an immediate impact on craving, the receptor side of the synapse, as well as stabilizing mood and energy levels. They are not intended to be a lifelong adjunct. A usual timeframe might be three to six months, with some people needing a longer time. After the body has resumed appropriate production, and the daily nutritional intake is appropriate, the regular use of amino acids should be discontinued as they have accomplished their job and are no longer needed. There may be periodic needs for additional supplement use based on stressful life situations.

There is material available to assist the counselor if they choose to integrate the use of supplements in their practice, or for persons in recovery who wish to use a more natural means to assist in their commitment to being clean and sober. The Bibliography lists several of these resources. In particular, the books authored by Charles Gant, MD, and Julia Ross, Ph.D., are exceptional references for further study. These resources provide guidelines regarding which products might be useful, the usual dosages, as well as some conditions to be aware of that might preclude their use.

CHAPTER 15

What about Children?

Especially if children come from a family where there is a history of substance dependence, they will be more at risk for early experimentation and consistent using. One of the most hopeful strategies for intervening successfully before excessive substance use is adopted as a lifestyle is ensuring balanced neurochemistry beginning with how we feed them.

Children need plenty of protein, especially at breakfast. Since protein is 'wake up' food, a tuna fish sandwich before they go to school, hard boiled eggs, cottage cheese, marinated and grilled chicken tenders (I think they are good cold), Salmon patties, mozzarella cheese sticks, tofu, egg salad sandwiches or smoothies will provide them with what they need to thrive. Cold cereal and packaged orange juice interfere with the ability to concentrate, stay focused on a task, or process information because they all fit into the category of 'go to sleep' foods.

Children under the age of ten can have an opposite effect to both caffeine and sugar. They can get a 'high' from the sugar, and a quieting effect from the caffeine. (The same is true for elders over sixty five). This is called paradoxical or idiosyncratic excitation. This is why we speak of children having a 'sugar high'. For them it acts like a stimulant and makes sitting still, paying attention, and staying focused on the task at hand difficult. It happens too frequently that they get sent off for an evaluation to see if they need medication for Attention Deficit issues.

For some children the diet change is enough - there just aren't Fruit Loops in the house anymore! Some parents have told me that the school teachers have noticed dramatic differences, other sibling's notice changes, the children are more fun to be with and there is less chaos in the home. Children at risk can also use some supplements if the diet change isn't enough. Here again, the experts will be helpful guides.

Children from families with an ancestry of alcohol dependence, or those suffering from lack of chemical balance, can often be helped by adding specific amino acids to their diet in dosages appropriate for their age.

EPILOGUE

From early human history we have always looked to others for comfort, assistance when we needed help, a sense of belonging, or healing when in pain. Cultures have evolved systems and designated healers to provide this function for the community. They were given a place of honor and regarded as essential in maintaining balance and well being for its members. They had an understanding that when the spirit was sick, the body began to show dis-ease and the community would then be affected by the individual's lack of wholeness.

Today we have healers that we also refer to with different titles who assume the responsibility of dealing with our pain. However, they may lack the same appreciation that a wounded spirit might be contributing to the physical conditions. As a result they tend to focus on their area of expertise for direction in prescribing relief.

We are an integrated whole and distress in one area causes distress in other parts of our being. As the reader hopefully can appreciate from the material that has been shared, the body affects the mind, emotions, and spirit. In turn, each of them has an impact on the body. To be a 'healer' means taking into consideration the wholeness of a human being and increasing our ability to be effective with the miracle of the person we are concerned about.

To each of you I send the warmest wishes for effectiveness in the work you do and a hug for being a gift to mankind.

BIBLIOGRAPHY

1. Amen, D., *Change Your Brain, Change Your Life.* New York: Random House. 1998.

2. Audette, Ray. *Neanderthin.* St. Martin's Paperbacks, NY. 1999.

3. Batmanghelidj, F., MD., *Your Body's Many Cries For Water.* Global Health Solutions, Inc. VA. 1997.

4. Batmanghelidj, F., MD., *You're Not Sick, You're Thirsty.* Warner Books. NY. 2003.

5. Blum, Kenneth, Ph.D., and Payne, James E., *Alcohol and the Addictive Brain,* The Free Press, NY. 1991.

6. Braverman, Erik R., MD., *The Edge Effect.* Sterling Publishing Co., Inc. NY. 2004.

7. Braverman, Eric. R., MD., *The Healing Nutrients Within.* Basic Health Publications. NJ. 2003.

8. Calbom, Cherie. *The Coconut Diet.* Warner Wellness, New York, NY. 2005.

9. Carper, Jean., *Your Miracle Brain.* HarperCollins Publisher, NY. 2000.

10. Chaitow, Leon, ND, DO., *Amino Acids in Therapy.* Thorson's Publishers, Inc., New York. 1985.

11. Enig, Mary G., *Know Your Fats*. Bethesda Press. Silver Spring, MD. 2000.

12. Erdmann, Robert, Ph.D., *The Amino Revolution*. Simon & Schuster, Inc., NY. 1987.

13. Fife, Bruce, CN, ND., *The Coconut Oil Miracle*. Penguin Group. New York, NY. 2004.

14. Fortuna, J., *Food, Brain Chemistry and Behavior*. Second Edition. Needham Heights, MA. Simon & Schuster. 1998.

15. Gant, Charles MD., and Lewis, Greg. Ph.D., *End Your Addiction Now*. SQUAREONE Publishers, Garden City Park, NY. 2010.

16. Hatherill, J. Robert., Ph.D., *The Brain Gate*. Lifeline Press. Washington, DC. 2003.

17. Jarvis, D. C., MD., *Folk Medicine*. Fawcett Books, NY. 1958.

18. Larson, Joan Matthews, Ph.D., *Seven Weeks to Sobriety*. Ballentine Publishing Group, NY. 1997.

19. Lesser, Michael, MD., *The Brain Chemistry Plan*. G. P. Putnam's Sons. NY. 2002.

20. Norden, M., *Beyond Prozac*. New York. HarperCollins. 1995.

21. Philpott, William H., MD, and Kalita, Dwight K., Ph.D. *Brain Allergies*. Keats Publishing. Lincolnwood, Illinois. 2000.

22. Restak, Richard, MD. (undated) *The Secret Life of the Brain*. Washington, DC. A co-publication of The DANA Press and Joseph Henry Press.

23. Ross, Julia, Ph.D., *The Diet Cure*. Penguin Putman, Inc., NY. 1999.

24. Ross, Julia, Ph.D., *The Mood Cure*, Penguin Group, New York, NY. 2002.

25. Sahelian, Ray, MD., *5-HTP, Nature's Serotonin Solution.* Avery Publishing Group, NY. 1998.

26. Sahley, Billie Jay, Ph.D. and Birkner, Katherine M., CRNA, Ph.D., *Heal With Amino Acids and Nutrients,* Pain & Stress Publications, San Antonio, Texas. 2000.

27. Stoll, Andrew L., *The Omega-3 Connection.* Simon & Schuster, New York, NY. 2001.

28. Vayda, William, DO., *Mood Foods.* Ulysses Press, Berkeley, CA. 1995.

29. Zull, James E., *The Art of Changing the Brain.* Sterling, Virginia. Stylus Publishing 2002.

ABOUT THE AUTHOR

Jean Armour has had an extensive career in the Human Services field as an instructor in a professional School of Nursing, a clinician and administrator in the mental health arena, an adjunct professor at the collegiate level, and as an administrator in the substance abuse field. She is now the Owner/Director of Armour Consulting, Inc. specializing in substance abuse related issues as a trainer, consultant, and clinical supervisor. Ms. Armour lives in Arvada, Colorado.

CPSIA information can be obtained
at www.ICGtesting.com
Printed in the USA
LVHW110333090419
613481LV00001B/52/P